Contents

INTRODUCTION

Far from being just another fad, The Fast Diet is a radical new way of thinking, your indispensable guide to simple and effective weight loss, without fuss or the need to endlessly deprive yourself.

If fasting interests you, The Fast Diet is a decent approach. It's going to take some serious willpower, but if you're up for the challenge, it can work. It's definitely not meant for everyone, so don't ignore the warnings.

Scientific trials have shown that intermittent fasting will help the pounds fly off and reduce your risk of diseases, including diabetes, cardiovascular disease, and even cancer, offering a dietary program you can incorporate into your busy daily life.

Dr Mosley's Fast Diet has become the health phenomenon of our times. And for good reason. This radical approach to weight loss really is as simple as it sounds. You eat normally for five days a week, then for just two days you cut your calorie intake (600 for men, 500 for women).

EVERYTHING YOU NEED TO KNOW ABOUT FASTING

Fasting is nothing new. In fact, we've all been doing it without even realising. Fasting, for most people, is the time between the last mouthful of food in the evening, and the first mouthful of food in the morning when we 'break the fast' at 'break-fast'. This type of fast normally lasts between 8 – 9 hours, depending on the times we eat. Recently, fasting for longer than this "normal" duration has increased in popularity, thanks to new science supporting the benefits associated with the technique.

As more diets have incorporated this method, it's made this type of dieting more mainstream but is it effective?

The 5:2 diet is a type of intermittent fasting which restricts energy intake on two of the seven days of the week. This is not a complete fast on those days. Instead, dieters usually consume around 1/4 of their normal intake. For ladies, this is typically around the 500-calorie mark, with men getting slightly more at 600 on the "fast" days. As calories are restricted on these days, the normal overnight fast is extended into the day, and this creates intermittent fasting.

The 5:2 Diet is not the only way to fast. Although incredibly popular, there is a new fasting diet that has grown in popularity due to its recent science-backed benefits. Although the name isn't as catchy, it's referred to as the "Restricted Eating Window Diet" (REWD). Although pretty self-explanatory, it basically restricts the length of time that we spend eating food each day, and increases the length of our overnight fast. It might sound similar to the 5:2 method, but for the REWD diet, there are no calorie restrictions. Research showed that when dieters ate within a restricted window of just 10-12 hours (instead of the usual 15) they ate up to 20% less calories, lost weight and became metabolically healthier.

Time limits applyFor the 5:2 diet, the "fast" window depends on when you have your first meal of the day. If you split your calories, the fast could last 15 hours, or if you power through until dinner, it could last for up to 22 hours. For REWD, the length and duration of the fast is up to you. However, you should aim for a minimum of 12–14 hours, and it is better to start the fast earlier in the evening rather than later. Looking at the pros and cons for both, the 5:2 diet gives you freedom with your eating habits on non-fast days, as you are only restricted on two days of the week. REWD has no limitations on what you can eat, but you do need to stay within your selected eating window, and do this for as many days of the week as possible. Choose what fits in better with your lifestyle.

Water is allowed when fastingFasting, by definition, is abstaining from food or drink, however, when it comes to fluids, we don't have to take this so literally. Fasting for specific religious reasons may include a restriction of all fluids, however on these particular fasting diets (REWD and 5:2), you are allowed to consume as much water as you like. During the fasting period of these diets you have to avoid all fruit juices, smoothies and even coffee, as all these contain energy or caffeine which has to be metabolised by the body. That being said, if you feel you can't function without your morning Starbucks, it's not the end of the world, just avoid drinks with added sugars and milks. Then, you can work towards eliminating these once your body gets used to longer fasts, transitioning to water.

Prepare to be hangryA disadvantage to eating this way is the hunger pangs you may experience in the first couple of weeks, in this instance, the hanger (hunger-anger) is real. For example, if you have pushed your breakfast back, reduced it or even eliminated it entirely, it may feel tougher in the morning as you are running on barely anything. When you're hungry, it's a natural instinct to grab something to eat. When you're fasting, whether it's a restriction of timings or calories, you need to train yourself to ignore the hunger pains. My tip would be to keep yourself busy so you have less opportunity to dwell on the fact you are hungry.

You can exercise whilst fasting It is suggested when following the 5:2 diet that on your low days you don't do a lot of vigorous exercise. There are two reasons for this, you will find the exercise tougher and feel more tired/depleted for the rest of the day. What I would suggest is you experiment with exercise on low days (on the 5:2) and during your fasting window (on the REWD). Yes, you may find it harder and you might become more hangry, however, you will soon learn when you're pushing yourself too far. I would suggest starting with lower intensity and shorter duration activities, then slowly increase. There are many benefits to exercising in a fasted state, but attempt it gradually and ease in.

There are multiple benefits of fastingThere are both mental and physical benefits to increasing the length of your fast. With regards to mental benefits, studies have shown that fasting diets are more sustainable than most diets, as they are a very simple way of dieting. You can either eat what you want, within an allotted time, or you can't go over a certain number of calories a couple of days a week. The physical advantages to fasting include weight loss, (due to the likely reduction in calories), increase cellular repair (which is stimulated in the fasted state), increased sensitivity to insulin, better sleep and a more diverse gut bacteria.

Practice makes perfect, Although simple, all dietary changes require time to adjust, so don't worry if it you bend the rules slightly at the beginning. An extra 50 calories or half an hour in the evening isn't going to ruin all you've worked for. Try setting yourself a target for the fast, sticking to eating well for five days a week, and then indulging in a treat meal at the weekend. It will allow you the freedom to enjoy all the social benefits food and drink offers (whether it's eating at a restaurant or going out to a bar and having a drink), without over-analysing, restricting or stressing out too much.

When you'll see changesLike all weight loss diets, you shouldn't become disheartened if you do not see changes immediately. However, you should start seeing and feeling some of the benefits mentioned in point eight as early as four weeks in. However, with dieting consistency is key, so I would suggest finding a partner to join you on the same diet. This means you have someone to motivate and be motivated by, as well as someone to vent your hanger with, but ultimately, someone to enjoy the benefits with

INTERMITTENT FASTING FOR BEGINNERS

Intermittent fasting involves cycling between periods of fasting and eating — and it's recently become very popular. Not only was it the "trendiest" weight loss search term in 2019, it was also prominently featured in a review article in The New England Journal of Medicine.

Intermittent fasting can provide significant health benefits if it is done right, including weight loss, reversal of type 2 diabetes and many other things. Plus, it can save you time and money. The goal of this beginner's guide is to provide everything you need to know about intermittent fasting, in order to get started.

Disclaimer: While intermittent fasting has many proven benefits, it's still controversial. A potential danger regards medications, especially for diabetes, where doses often need to be adapted. Discuss any changes in medication and relevant lifestyle changes with your doctor.

This guide is written for adults with health issues, including obesity that could benefit from intermittent fasting. People who should not fast include those who are underweight or have eating disorders like anorexia, women who are pregnant or breastfeeding, and people under the age of 18.

Intermittent fasting – isn't that starvation?

No. Fasting differs from starvation in one crucial way: control. Starvation is the involuntary absence of food for a long time. This can lead to severe suffering or even death. It is neither deliberate nor controlled.

On the other hand, fasting is the voluntary avoidance of food for spiritual, health, or other reasons. It's done by someone who is not underweight and has enough stored body fat to live off. When done correctly, fasting should not cause suffering, and certainly never death.

Food is easily available, but you choose not to eat it. This can be for any period of time, from a few hours up to a few days or with medical supervision even a week or more. You may begin a fast at any time of your choosing, and you may end a fast at will too.

Anytime you are not eating, you are intermittently fasting.4For example, you may fast between dinner and breakfast the next day, a period of approximately 12-14 hours. In that sense, intermittent fasting should be considered a part of everyday life.

It is perhaps the oldest and most powerful dietary intervention imaginable.

Consider the term "break fast." This refers to the meal that breaks your fast – which is done daily.

Rather than being some sort of cruel and unusual punishment, the English language implicitly acknowledges that fasting should be performed daily, even if only for a short duration.

Intermittent fasting is not something unusual but a part of everyday, normal life. It is perhaps the oldest and most powerful dietary intervention imaginable.6 Yet somehow we have missed its power and overlooked its therapeutic potential.

INTERMITTENT FASTING FOR WEIGHT LOSS

Balancing eating and fasting

At its very core, intermittent fasting simply allows the body to use its stored energy, by burning off excess body fat. It is important to realize that this is normal and humans have evolved to fast for shorter time periods – hours or days – without detrimental health consequences. Body fat is merely food energy that has been stored away. If you don't eat, your body will simply "eat" its own fat for energy.

Life is about balance. The good and the bad, the yin and the yang. The same applies to eating and fasting. Fasting, after all, is simply the flip side of eating. If you are not eating, you are fasting.

Here's how it works:

When we eat, more food energy is ingested than can immediately be used. Some of this energy must be stored away for later use. Insulin is the key hormone involved in the storage of food energy. Insulin rises when we eat, helping to store the excess energy in two separate ways. Carbohydrates are broken down into individual glucose (sugar) units, which can be linked into long chains to form glycogen, which is then stored in the liver or muscle.

There is, however, very limited storage space for carbohydrates; and once that is reached, the liver starts to turn the excess glucose into fat. This process is called de-novo lipogenesis (meaning literally "making new fat").

Some of this newly created fat is stored in the liver, but most of it is exported to other fat deposits in the body. While this is a more complicated process, there is almost no limit to the amount of fat that can be created. So, two complementary food energy storage systems exist in our bodies. One is easily accessible but with limited storage space (glycogen), and the other is more difficult to access but has almost unlimited storage space (body fat).

The process goes in reverse when we do not eat. Insulin levels fall, signaling the body to start burning stored energy because no more is coming through food. Blood glucose falls, so the body must now pull glucose out of storage to burn for energy. Glycogen is the most easily accessible energy source. It is broken down into glucose molecules to provide energy for the body's other cells. This can provide enough energy to power much of the body's needs for 24-36 hours. After that, the body will primarily be breaking down fat for energy.

So the body only really exists in two states – the fed state and the fasted state. Either we are storing food energy (increasing stores), or we are burning stored energy (decreasing stores). It's one or the other. If eating and fasting are balanced, then there should be no net weight change.

If we start eating the minute we roll out of bed and do not stop until we go to sleep, we spend almost all our time in the fed state. Over time, we may gain weight because we have not allowed our body any time to burn stored food energy.

To restore balance or to lose weight, we may simply need to increase the amount of time spent burning food energy.That's intermittent fasting. In essence, intermittent fasting allows the body to use its stored energy. The important thing to understand is that there is nothing wrong with that. That is how our bodies are designed. That's what dogs, cats, lions and bears do. That's what humans do.

If you're eating every third hour, as is often recommended, then your body will constantly use the incoming food energy. It may not need to burn much body fat, if any. You may just be storing fat.14 Your body may be saving it for a time when there is nothing to eat. If this happens, you lack balance. You lack intermittent fasting.

INTERMITTENT FASTING BENEFITS

Intermittent fasting's most obvious benefit is weight loss. However, there are many potential benefits beyond this, some of which have been known since ancient times.

The fasting periods were often called 'cleanses,' 'detoxifications' or 'purifications,' but the idea is similar – to abstain from eating food for a certain period of time. People believed that this period of abstinence from food would clear their systems of toxins and rejuvenate them.

Some of the purported health benefits of intermittent fasting include:

• Weight and body fat loss

• Increased fat burning

• Lowered blood insulin and sugar levels

• Possibly reversal of type 2 diabetes

- Possibly improved mental clarity and concentration

- Possibly increased energy

- Possibly increased growth hormone, at least in the short term

- Possibly an improved blood cholesterol profile

- Possibly longer life

- Possibly activation of cellular cleansing by stimulating autophagy

- Possibly reduction of inflammation

In addition, fasting offers many important unique advantages that are not available in typical diets.

While diets can complicate life, intermittent fasting may simplify it. While diets can take time, fasting saves time. While diets may be limited in their availability, fasting is available anywhere. Here are even more reasons to try it, along with more details: The 7 practical benefits of intermittent fasting

INTERMITTENT FASTING RESULTS

Intermittent fasting: down 42 pounds in 14 months

Intermittent fasting offers plenty of flexibility. You can fast for as long or short as you like, but fasts longer than a few days may require medical supervision.30 Here are some popular regimens. Generally, shorter fasts are done more frequently.

16:8

This way of doing intermittent fasting involves daily fasting for 16 hours. Sometimes this is also referred to as an 8-hour eating 'window.' You eat all your meals within an 8-hour time period and fast for the remaining 16 hours. Generally, this is done daily or almost daily.

For example, you may eat all your meals within the time period of 11:00 am and 7:00 pm. Generally, this means skipping breakfast, but some people prefer to skip dinner instead. Typically this involves eating either two or three meals within this 8-hour period.

20:4

This involves a 4-hour eating window and a 20-hour fast. For example, you might eat between 2:00 pm and 6:00 pm every day and fast for the other 20 hours. This would involve eating either one large, lengthy meal or two smaller meals within this period.

Longer fasts (>24 hours)

24-hour fasts

This way of doing intermittent fasting involves fasting from dinner to dinner (or lunch to lunch). If you eat dinner on day 1, you would skip the next day's breakfast and lunch and eat dinner again on day 2. This is also known as "one meal a day," or OMAD. It is generally done two to three times per week.

5:2 fast

This is the version of intermittent fasting that has the most scientific support, as most studies on intermittent fasting have featured similar advice. The 5:2 fast involves five regular eating days and two fasting days. However, on these two fasting days, you are allowed to eat 500 calories on each day. These calories can be consumed at any time during the day – either spread throughout the day or as a single meal.

Alternate-day fasting

Another related approach to 5:2 is to have "fasting" days with 500 calories not just twice a week, but every other day.

36-hour fasts

This involves fasting for the entire day. For example, if you eat dinner on day 1, you would fast for all of day 2 and not eat again until breakfast on day 3. This is generally 36 hours of fasting. This might provide a more powerful weight-loss benefit and may help avoid the temptation to overeat dinner on day 2.

However, there are some risks involved with fasting more than 24 hours.

Extended fasting

The first rule of extended fasts is to always check with your health care provider to ensure you are not at risk for fasting complications.

Generally, for fasts greater than 48 hours, I recommend a multivitamin to avoid micronutrient deficiency. The world record for fasting is 382 days (although we don't recommend this!), and going 7-14 days may be possible for some people.

I discourage people from fasting for more than 14 days due to high risk of refeeding syndrome, a dangerous shift in fluids and minerals that can occur when food is re-introduced after a long fast.

Who should NOT fast?

You should not do intermittent fasting if you are:

• Underweight (BMI < 18.5) or have an eating disorder like anorexia.

• Pregnant – you need extra nutrients for your child.

• Breastfeeding – you need extra nutrients for your child.

• A child under 18 – you need extra nutrients to grow.

• You can probably fast, but may need medical supervision, under these conditions:

• If you have diabetes mellitus type 1 or type 2.

• If you take prescription medication.

• If you have gout or high uric acid.

• If you have any serious medical conditions, such as liver disease, kidney disease, or heart disease.

Won't intermittent fasting put me into starvation mode?

Not likely. This is the most common myth about intermittent fasting, and generally it's not true. In fact, some studies indicate that intermittent fasting may even increase the basal metabolic rate (at least initially) and might potentially improve overall body composition.

Can I exercise during fasting?

Yes. You can continue all your usual activities, including exercise, while fasting. You do not need to eat before exercising to provide energy.38 Instead, your body can burn stored energy (like body fat) for fuel. However, for long-duration aerobic exercise, eating before exercise may increase performance. It's also important to drink fluids and replenish sodium (salt) around exercise when fasting. This is good to know if you're competing.

POSSIBLE SIDE EFFECTS

There can be a number of possible side effects of intermittent fasting. Here's what to do if you encounter them:

Hunger is the most common side effect of intermittent fasting. This may be less of an issue if you're already on a keto or low-carb, higher-fat diet.

Constipation is common. Less going in means less going out. However, keep in mind this is a normal response to eating less. It is not a concern and shouldn't require treatment unless you experience significant bloating or abdominal discomfort. Standard laxatives or magnesium supplements can be used, if needed.

Headaches are common and tend to disappear after the first few times on fasts. Taking some extra salt often helps mitigate such headaches.

Mineral water may help if your stomach tends to gurgle.

Other possible side effects include dizziness, heartburn and muscle cramps.

A more serious side effect is the refeeding syndrome. Fortunately, this is rare and generally only happens with extended fasts (5-10 days or more) when one is undernourished.

Since most of these side effects are manageable, they do not mean you have to stop your fast. However, if you truly feel unwell, are excessively dizzy, profoundly weak or have other severe symptoms, then you should break your fast.

Just remember to go slowly when you break it and prioritize fluids and salt (bone broth is a great way to start). And of course, if the symptoms persist, see your doctor immediately.

Fortunately, severe side effects are very rare, especially if you remain hydrated and supplement with electrolytes.

QUESTIONS TO ASK WHEN YOU START FAST DIET

Why does my blood sugar go up during fasting?

While this does not happen with everyone, it can occur due to hormonal changes that occur during intermittent fasting. Your body is producing sugar in order to provide energy for your system. This is a variation of the dawn phenomenon and in general is not a concern as long as blood sugars are not elevated the rest of the day.

How do I manage hunger?

The most important thing to realize is that hunger usually passes like a wave. Many people worry that hunger during intermittent fasting will continue to build until it is intolerable, but this does not normally happen.46 Instead, hunger comes in a wave. If you simply ignore it and drink a cup of tea or coffee, it will often pass.

During extended fasts, hunger will often increase into the second day. After that, it gradually recedes, and many people report a complete loss of hunger sensation by day 3 or 4. Your body is now being powered by fat. In essence, your body is 'eating' its own fat for breakfast, lunch and dinner and therefore is no longer hungry.

Won't intermittent fasting burn muscle?

That depends on the person and the duration of the fast. During fasting, the body first breaks down glycogen into glucose for energy. After that, the body increases body fat breakdown to provide energy. Excess amino acids (the building blocks of proteins) are also used for energy, but the body does not burn its own muscle for fuel unless it has to.

Some studies, however, suggest that leaner individuals are at higher risk of lean body mass loss, and even reduced metabolic rate. Yet it appears this is less of a concern with overweight subjects. In my experience with over 1,000 patients on various intermittent fasting regimens, I have not yet seen a single case of significant muscle loss.

What are your top tips for intermittent fasting?

Here are the seven top tips, briefly:

• Drink water.

• Stay busy.

• Drink coffee or tea.

• Ride out the hunger waves.

• Give yourself one month to see if intermittent fasting (such as 16:8) is a good fit for you.

• Follow a low-carb diet between fasting periods. This reduces hunger and makes intermittent fasting easier. It may also increase the effect on weight loss and type 2 diabetes reversal, etc.

• Don't binge after fasting

How do I break a fast?

Eating too large a meal after fasting (a mistake that we have ALL done, myself included) can give you a stomach ache. While this is hardly serious, people usually learn quickly to eat as normally as possible after a fast.

Isn't it important to have breakfast every morning?

Not necessarily. This appears to be an old misconception, based on speculation and statistics, and it does not hold up when it's tested. Skipping your morning meal gives your body more time to burn fat for energy. Since hunger is lowest in the morning, it may be easiest to skip it and break your fast later in the day.

Can women fast?

Yes, but there are exceptions. Women who are underweight, pregnant or breastfeeding should not fast.

Furthermore, for women trying to conceive, be aware that – perhaps especially for athletic women with low body fat percentage – intermittent fasting might increase the risk of irregular menses, and lower the chance of conception.

Other than that, there is no special reason why women should not fast. Women can have problems during intermittent fasting, but so can men. Sometimes women do not get the results they want, but that happens to men, too. Studies show that the average weight loss for women and men who fast is similar.

Isn't fasting the same as reducing calories?

No, not necessarily. Fasting can reduce the time you spend eating and primarily addresses the question of "when to eat."62 Calorie reduction addresses the question of "what and how much to eat." They are separate issues and should not be confused with each other.

Now that you know more about intermittent fasting, how do you get started;

Decide what type of fast you want to do.

Decide upon the length of time you want to fast.

Start fasting. If you do not feel well, or if you have any concerns, then stop.

Continue all your usual activities outside of eating. Stay busy and live normally. Imagine you're "eating" a full meal of your own fat.

Break the fast gently.

Repeat.

Yes, it can be that simple.

WHAT YOU NEED TO KNOW ABOUT OMAD

OMAD an abbreviation for One Meal A Day is a popular pattern of eating many are using to lose weight or improve metabolic health. But is it a healthy and sustainable way to lose weight? And is it a healthy long-term lifestyle?

Simply put, OMAD means eating one meal in a day. It doesn't specify what you eat, or even what time you eat. It simply directs you to eat once. OMAD is the longest form of time-restricted eating, equivalent to a 23:1 fast (fasting for 23 hours and eating in a 1-hour window). In its purest sense, OMAD doesn't dictate calorie restriction or specific macronutrient composition. That said, we encourage you to continue your healthy, low-carb diet at that meal. And be sure to keep reading to the end for other practical tips for eating OMAD.

The one meal a day (OMAD) diet is, simply put, fasting from food for 23 hours a day and eating whatever you'd like for one meal. That meal can range from a double cheeseburger and fries to a more healthful salad loaded with greens, roasted veggies, whole grains, beans, nuts, and seeds. The idea is by limiting your calorie consumption throughout the day, you can feast on one meal (usually defined as a one-hour window) and still lose weight. Water and unsweetened coffee and tea are allowed, but otherwise, the kitchen is closed — all day long.

Is the OMAD diet the same as intermittent fasting?

The one meal a day diet is a type of time-restricted intermittent fasting, in which dieters will fast for 12 or more hours per day. In this case, of course, it's 23. Most people do this by starting a fast at night, skipping breakfast, and eating their first meal in the middle of the day — with another seven hours or so left to fantasize about food before going to bed.

Can you lose weight by eating one meal a day?

When you're only eating one meal per day, you're likely consuming a significantly fewer amount of calories than you normally would. Reduced calorie consumption usually results in weight loss; larger-scale studies have found that people who practiced fasting and people who simply decreased calorie intake overall lost the same amount of weight.

It's very easy to feel deprived when practicing the OMAD diet, which could lead to binging and falling off the wagon. Prolonged periods of restriction often beget weight cycling (i.e., "yo-yo-dieting") and changes to your hunger hormones and metabolism. Ultimately, you may feel hungrier after trying the one meal a day diet than you might've felt before you started this restrictive plan. To make food choices that ultimately lead to better health and subsequent weight loss, it's not feasible for many of us to simply restrict food entirely for set periods of time.

Is the OMAD diet healthy?

The idea behind intermittent fasting is that its gives your vital organs, digestive hormones, and metabolic functions a "break" and reduces oxidative stress on the body. Proponents believe reducing stress via fasting improves the function of your organ tissues, reduces inflammation, and lowers your risk for chronic disease. It's also credited with reducing susceptibility to insulin resistance, which could lower your risk for diabetes. However, there's substantial evidence suggesting that any benefit is quickly undone as soon as you break the fast, causing the appetite-suppressing hormones to switch gears and make you feel even hungrier than you felt at baseline.

A real potential benefit of time-restricted fasting is that it could help you go to bed earlier — a very crucial component to any weight loss plan. Getting seven hours of sleep per night as been linked to weight management, reduced risk of chronic disease, and improved metabolic benefits.

Is the OMAD diet bad for you?

There's very little scientific data supporting the one meal a day diet, which is scarily similar to a disordered eating practice. There are some major risks and potential negative consequences associated with this type of pattern:

You're ignoring your body's own hunger cues. If you've only got one hour out of the day to consume nutrients, it's highly likely that you're going to eat as much as you possibly can, which isn't exactly priming your body and intuition to understand when you feel full or hungry.

You could miss out on important nutrients. In order to get enough key antioxidants, minerals, and phytonutrients, you'd have to pack in five daily servings of veggies and fruit, not to mention whole grains, legumes, nuts, seeds, lean protein, and some dairy products (or dairy alternatives) in that one-hour window.

Your bad cholesterol levels could go up. Fasting has been linked to increases in LDL cholesterol, which is basically the opposite of what you're trying to achieve!

You could slow your metabolism. The more you restrict, the slower your metabolism becomes as a response. That can lead to unwanted side effects in the long run, including weight gain.

What happens if you only eat one meal a day?

The side effects of restricting food for nearly an entire day can include:

• Lightheadedness

• Nausea

• Blood pressure destabilization

• Dizziness

- Confusion

- Hypoglycemia (low blood sugar)

- Dehydration

Consider what else might happen by eating one meal per day. It's hard to exercise regularly (another important factor to your health) when you're not fueled appropriately. You could miss out on various experiences and meals shared with family and friends. Plus, you're following rules instead of making choices. That's the opposite of cultivating a mindful eating practice, which could majorly backfire when you decide to go off of this plan.

The Bottom Line

If you still want to try the OMAD diet, strive for a wide variety of nutrient-rich foods like fruits, veggies, whole grains, and lean proteins. Do not try this type of plan if you're pregnant, lactating, or taking medication that requires food for metabolism of the drug. Even if you don't experience any short-term side effects, studies have yet to find out how fasting can affect humans in the long run.

Instead, I'd encourage you to keep it as simple as possible: Experiment with an "early bird special" for dinner; close your kitchen once you're finished; aim to get more sleep overnight, and sit down for a full breakfast at your usual time tomorrow.

BENEFITS OF OMAD

clinical experience

Clinicians experienced in prescribing intermittent fasting and low-carb nutrition frequently use OMAD as a tool to help with weight loss stalls. When a patient is eating low carb but isn't losing weight as expected, temporary use of OMAD can help kick-start weight loss. You can read more about addressing weight loss stalls in our evidence-based guide.

Many who eat in an OMAD pattern do so for the ease of only preparing food and eating once each day. This can be especially helpful for those who travel frequently, those who perform shift work, and those with hectic and busy schedules.

Think about how much time you spend planning, shopping for, and preparing meals. (And we haven't even mentioned dealing with dirty dishes.) If you eat three meals per day, how much time could you save by cutting that by two-thirds? As a form of time-restricted eating and intermittent fasting, OMAD may help reduce hyperinsulinemia, control diabetes and improve metabolic syndrome. Consistent clinical experience shows that widening the fasting window can help improve these metabolic conditions. So, when used appropriately, OMAD could potentially deliver better results than shorter fasts.

Some see OMAD as an "easy" way to reduce calorie intake. When you only allow yourself to eat in a 30-to-60-minute time window, it is physically difficult to exceed your daily calorie needs. It's not impossible (just ask hot dog speed-eating champion Joey Chestnut, who can eat more than 10,000 calories in 10 minutes) but it sure is challenging. For those who benefit from a firm schedule that restricts snacking, OMAD can be the strategy that works best. (Of course, "easy" is in the eye of the beholder!)

Eating disorders

Any eating pattern that promotes a cycle of food restriction followed by extra food consumption can trigger disordered eating behavior in susceptible people. So if you have a history of eating disorders, you should probably avoid OMAD.

Chronic caloric restriction

Creating an environment where you naturally reduce caloric intake is one of the clinical benefits of OMAD. The other side of that coin is that it can be difficult to obtain adequate calories if eating OMAD long term on a daily basis. OMAD can then start to look a lot like chronic caloric restriction. Although chronic caloric restriction helps with initial weight loss, it poses long-term concerns because it tends to lower resting metabolic rate, which makes weight loss very difficult to maintain.

Inadequate protein intake

Just as OMAD promotes caloric restriction, it can also lead to protein restriction. Since protein helps you feel full and satisfied, it can be difficult to eat your entire daily requirement in one sitting.4The average 5'10," 81-kg male should eat about 110 grams of protein daily (read more about how much protein we should eat). If you can eat a 16-oz ribeye plus a couple of fried eggs in one sitting, then it may not be a concern. But if that sounds like a lot to you, then your protein intake may be too low with daily OMAD.

Excessive carb intake

If you are trying to consistently remain in ketosis, we recommend restricting net carb intake to less than 20 grams per day. But in general, we also advise that you spread out your carb intake so each meal has no more than 10 grams. With OMAD, you eat only one meal, so you could theoretically eat all 20 grams of carbs in one sitting. While that is still compatible with a keto diet, those who are highly insulin resistant may respond to a 20-gram carb load with glucose and insulin spikes.

GI upset and diarrhea

Some find the consistent cycle of no food followed by a large amount of food causes abdominal discomfort and even diarrhea. Although it's hard to estimate how many OMAD eaters experience this, our clinical expert panel considers it uncommon but not unheard of.

Taking medications with food

For those who need to take prescription medications with food more than once per day, OMAD presents a significant hurdle. If this is the case for you, discuss with your healthcare provider if other options exist. If not, then OMAD is likely not safe for you.

Exercise

Some people find it difficult to exercise while fasting. If you are active, this would make following an OMAD pattern challenging. However, we encourage you to at least try fasted exercise, as some findings suggest that it may help with weight and fat loss (although the literature is inconclusive on this point).

WARNING SIGNS

Many people do well, even thrive, with time-restricted eating and intermittent fasting. Others are more susceptible to side effects. Feeling a little hungry and a little low in energy are expected. But feeling unwell, extremely fatigued, dizzy, nauseated, or having other severe side effects are abnormal responses to intermittent fasting and OMAD. If you experience any of these severe side effects, OMAD is likely not the best choice for you. You can work with your doctor to determine if any changes (like greater adaptation to low carb and shorter fasting regimens) could make it an option in the future.

WHAT SCIENCE SAYS

The science on intermittent fasting and time-restricted eating is growing, seemingly on a weekly basis. The problem is that different studies investigate different protocols. For instance, one recent study showed that a 14:10 time-restricted eating pattern can promote weight loss and metabolic health. How do we know if these benefits occur with OMAD? If 14:10 is helpful, is 23:1 better? It might be. If lowering insulin levels and mobilizing fat stores for 14 hours is beneficial, it makes sense that doing it for 23 hours could be even more so. Yet this assumes that a longer time frame doesn't introduce any counterbalancing, negative effects.

Other studies suggest longer fasting windows have a net benefit, although none capture OMAD eating perfectly. For instance, another trial showed that in obese patients with diabetes, two weeks of eating within a 7-hour window (17 hours of fasting) reduced fasting and postprandial blood glucose more than eating within a 13-hour eating window (11 hrs of fasting).

Closer to a standard OMAD, a 2009 crossover study compared eating 3 meals per day to eating the exact same food allotment in a 20:4 eating window. The diet was 15% protein, 35% fat and 50% carbs. During the 8-week period of eating within a 4-hour window, participants lost 4.4 pounds (2 kg) of body fat while maintaining their lean mass. By contrast, they lost no weight or fat while eating three meals per day. In addition, immediately after the time-restricted eating portion of the study, patients had lower triglycerides (93 vs 102 mg/dL), higher HDL (63 vs 56 mg/dL), and higher LDL (136 vs 113 mg/dL).

While the authors warned about the higher LDL, looking further we see that the total cholesterol-to-HDL radio remained the same after both diets at 3.4, and the TG:HDL ratio improved in the time-restricted eating group (1.5 vs 1.8). Therefore, even though LDL went up, overall lipid profiles improved during time-restricted eating.

Interestingly, the subjects reported increased hunger throughout the time they ate within a 4-hour window. But keep in mind this was a high-carbohydrate diet. Would it have been different on a low-carb diet? Clinical experience suggests that yes, they would have been less hungry, but we don't have comparative data.

So, it seems reasonable to extrapolate this data to OMAD, and predict that it may also provide the same or greater benefits. But we still don't know if the benefit remains for long-term, daily OMAD. Since we have hesitation about the daily use of OMAD, the lack of long-term data is concerning. That is where alternate-day fasting comes in.

Alternate-day fasting is essentially every-other-day OMAD. Eat normally for a day, then follow the OMAD pattern for a day. This addresses concerns about chronic caloric restriction because every other day is "normal" eating, alternating with a fasting or calorie-restricted day. One study compared ADF to chronic caloric restriction and found it was better tolerated and delivered similar benefits for weight loss and body composition. Another study in patients with type 2 diabetes showed that one day of consuming 500 calories followed by two days of normal eating produced HbA1c improvements similar to those observed during chronic caloric restriction.

While none of these studies definitively show OMAD is healthy and sustainable, we can reasonably extrapolate from the data and suggest that OMAD can likely be a part of a healthy, sustainable eating proto

BEST USE OF OMAD

OMAD appears to be a powerful tool to help with weight loss and metabolic health. That said, we caution against chronic daily use of OMAD for all the reasons outlined above. Instead, for those who may benefit from more pronounced time-restricted eating, using OMAD one to three times per week, on non-consecutive days, could be an effective tool. This is not a science-based protocol with plenty of high-quality evidence, but is instead based on the information presented in this guide and on clinical experience.

Just remember, OMAD is not a license to eat whatever you want. What you eat for your one meal still matters. We recommend you stick with your low-carb plan on OMAD and non-OMAD days alike. In fact, clinical experience suggests that a well-formulated low-carb diet makes intermittent fasting and OMAD easier to do by reducing hunger and cravings. So, you can consider LCHF as your secret weapon to build your OMAD superpower.

Here is a sample week utilizing OMAD:

Monday: eat two meals with 16:8 time-restricted eating, targeting 1,800 calories.

Tuesday: OMAD, around 1,200 calories (assuming a standard 1,800-calorie intake). Aim for 30% protein (105 grams), 10 grams carbs and 104 grams fat. Some may find this volume challenging. If so, consider lengthening your eating window so that you eat a "snack" of nuts and cheese and then, an hour later, eat your full meal.

Wednesday: eat two meals with 16:8 time-restricted eating, 1,800 calories

Thursday: OMAD, similar to Tuesday

Friday: eat two meals with 16:8 time-restricted eating, 1,800 calories

Saturday: free day to eat how your social schedule dictates (just stay on your low-carb plan!)

Sunday: OMAD, similar to Tuesday

OMAD meal plan

A week of OMAD

OMAD is short for "One Meal a Day" and it's an increasingly popular way of doing time-restricted eating or intermittent fasting. This meal plan helps you do it in a safe and effective way, ensuring you get enough calories and protein each day while helping you meet your low-carb and weight loss goals. The plan has you alternating OMAD one day followed by two meals, lunch and dinner, the next day. It is simple and no fuss. And you'll be eating delicious, nourishing meals. Do make sure you drink lots of water (tea or black coffee is fine, too.) And get enough salt to minimize side effects like headaches and keto flu.

WHAT YOU SHOULD KNOW ABOUT THE 16:8 DIET BEFORE YOU START FASTING

This popular weight-loss method can backfire if you're not careful. Silicon Valley moguls, celebrities, and social media influencers alike prescribe to the 16:8 diet, a form of intermittent fasting also known as the 8-hour diet. Proponents claim that restricting mealtimes — you eat during an 8-hour window each day and fast the rest of the time — helps with everything from weight loss to lowering the risk of chronic disease. The problem with this popular method is that you're not making decisions based on how full or hungry you feel, but rather on a restricted time window — a setup that can backfire in the long run if you're not careful. Here's what you need to know about 16:8 fasting before you start missing meals.

TYPES OF INTERMITTENT FASTING AND WHAT TO KNOW ABOUT THEM

The diet approach is growing in popularity as a way to possibly lose weight, stave off disease, and boost longevity. But there are several different ways to do it, depending on your lifestyle and goals.

The Proposed Health Benefits of Intermittent Fasting

When it comes to weight loss, there are two thoughts behind why IF has the potential to work. The first: "Periods of fasting produce a net calorie deficit, and so you lose weight. The other concept is more complex: This approach may prevent what's called the "plateau phenomenon" from happening.

You may remember the famous, so-called Biggest Loser study, published in August 2016 in the journal Obesity. The researchers followed up with participants after six years, and despite the initial impressive weight loss, they regained most of the weight, and their metabolic rates had slowed, such that they burned far fewer calories than would have been expected.

Though more research is needed on the safety and effectiveness of IF, one of the touted benefits of this approach is it may prevent this metabolic sputtering. "Most people who try diet and exercise to lose weight tend to fall off the wagon and regain weight. Hormones that promote weight regain, like hunger hormones, are kicked into full gear, and the thought is that IF may be a way to prevent this metabolic adaptation from happening," says Dr. Kumar. Normal periods of eating in IF "trick" your body into losing weight before the plateau happens.

So, does it actually lead to weight loss? Anecdotal evidence has led proponents of the plan to concur with a resounding yes. "For the people who can adhere to IF, it does work," says Kumar. But fans of the approach claim there's so much more to IF than just a lean body.

WHO SHOULDN'T TRY INTERMITTENT FASTING

Not everyone should (or needs to) try IF. A few groups who shouldn't: women who are pregnant or trying to become pregnant (extended fasting periods may throw off your menstrual cycle), those taking diabetes medication (blood sugar can drop too far in the absence of food), or anyone on multiple drugs (food, or lack of it, can affect absorption and dosage), says Kumar. Also, if you have a history of eating disorders, introducing periods where you're "not allowed" to eat can put you on a dangerous path to a relapse.

Know that IF has some side effects. You may be cranky "hanger" is real during fasting periods because low blood sugar can mess with your mood. You also still need to have a healthy diet when you do eat. "One thought is that it would be difficult to make up a calorie deficit if you fasted for two days, but in our society with access to calorie-dense items, you could probably do it, Focus on balanced, nutrient-packed choices, like fruits, vegetables, lean meats, legumes, and whole grains (though some experts, like Dr. Shemek, also pair IF with low-carb or keto styles of eating). Expect that for the first couple of weeks you may deal with lower energy, bloating, and cravings until your body adjusts, says Shemek.

TYPES OF INTERMITTENT FASTING TO CONSIDER

There are so many different ways to do IF, and that's a great thing. If this is something you're interested in doing, you can find the type that will work best for your lifestyle, which increases the chances of success. Here are seven:

5:2 Fasting

This is one of the most popular IF methods. The idea is to eat normally for five days (don't count calories) and then on the other two eat 500 or 600 calories a day for women and men, respectively. The fasting days are any days of your choosing.

The idea is that short bouts of fasting keep you compliant; should you be hungry on a fast day, you just have to look forward to tomorrow when you can "feast" again. "Some people say 'I can do anything for two days, but it's too much to cut back on what I eat all seven days,'" says Kumar. For these people, a 5:2 approach may work for them over calorie cutting across the entire week.

That said, the authors of The Fast Diet advise against making fast days on days where you may be doing a lot of endurance exercise. If you're prepping for a bike or running race (or run high-mileage weeks), evaluate if this type of fasting could work with your training plan or speak with a sports nutritionist.

Time-Restricted Fasting

With this type of IF, you choose an eating window every day, which should ideally leave a 14 to 16 hour fast. (Due to hormonal concerns, Shemek recommends that women fast for no more than 14 hours daily.) "Fasting promotes autophagy, the natural 'cellular housekeeping' process where the body clears debris and other things that stand in the way of the health of mitochondria, which begins when liver glycogen is depleted, Doing this may help maximize fat cell metabolism and helps optimize insulin function, she says.

For this to work, you may set your eating window from 9 a.m. to 5 p.m., for instance. This can work especially well for someone with a family who eats an early dinner anyway, says Kumar. Then much of the time spent fasting is time spent sleeping anyway. (You also don't technically have to "miss" any meals, depending on when you set your window.) But this is dependent on how consistent you can be. If your schedule is frequently changing, or you need or want the freedom to go out to breakfast occasionally, head out for a late date night, or go to happy hour, daily periods of fasting may not be for you.

Overnight Fasting

This approach is the simplest of the bunch and involves fasting for a 12-hour period every day. For example: Choose to stop eating after dinner by 7 p.m. and resume eating at 7 a.m. with breakfast the next morning. Autophagy does still happen at the 12-hour mark, though you'll get more mild cellular benefits. This is the minimum number of fasting hours she recommends.

A pro of this method is that it's easy to implement. Also, you don't have to skip meals; if anything, all you're doing is eliminating a bedtime snack (if you ate one to begin with). But this method doesn't maximize the advantages of fasting. If you're using fasting for weight loss, a smaller fasting window means more time to eat, and it may not help you decrease the number of calories you consume.

Eat Stop Eat

This approach was developed by author Brad Pilon in his book Eat Stop Eat: The Shocking Truth That Makes Weight Loss Simple Again. His approach differs from other plans in that he stresses flexibility. Simply put, he stresses that fasting is just taking a break from food for a time. You complete one or two 24-hour fasts per week and commit to a resistance training program. "When your fast is over, I want you to pretend that it never happened and eat responsibly. That's it. Nothing else," he says on his website.

Eating responsibly refers to going back to a normal way of eating where you don't binge because you just fasted, but you also don't restrict yourself with an extreme diet or eating less than you need. Occasional fasting combined with regular weight training is best for fat loss. By going on one or two 24-hour fasts during the week, you allow yourself to eat a slightly higher amount of calories on the other five or six no fasting days. That, he says, makes it easier and more enjoyable to end the week in a calorie deficit without feeling as if you had to be on an extreme diet.

Whole-Day Fasting

Here, you eat once a day. Some people choose to eat dinner and then not eat again until the next day's dinner. That means your fasting period is 24 hours. This differs from the 5:2 method. Fasting periods are essentially 24 hours (dinner to dinner or lunch to lunch), whereas with 5:2 the fasting is actually 36 hours. (For example, you eat dinner on Sunday, "fast" Monday by eating 500 to 600 calories, and break it with breakfast on Tuesday.)

The advantage is that, if done for weight loss, it's really tough (though not impossible) to eat an entire day's worth of calories in one sitting. The disadvantage to this approach is that it's hard to get all the nutrients your body needs to function optimally with just one meal. Not to mention, this approach is tough to stick to. You might get really hungry by the time dinner rolls around, and that can lead you to consume not-so-great, calorie-dense choices. Think about it: When you're ravenous, you're not exactly craving broccoli. Many people also drink coffee in excess to get through their hunger, says Shemek, which can have negative effects on your sleep. You may also notice brain fog throughout the day if you're not eating.

Alternate-Day Fasting

This approach was popularized by Krista Varady, PhD, a nutrition professor at the University of Illinois in Chicago. People might fast every other day, with a fast consisting of 25 percent of their calorie needs (about 500 calories) and no fasting days being normal eating days. This is a popular approach for weight loss. In fact, a small study published in Nutrition Journal by Dr. Varady and colleagues found that alternate day fasting was effective in helping obese adults lose weight. The side effects (like hunger) decreased by week two and the participants started feeling more satisfied on the diet after week four.

The downside is that during the eight weeks in the experiment, participants said that they were never really "full," which can make adhering to this approach challenging.

Choose-Your-Day Fasting

This is more of a choose-your-own adventure. You might do the time-restricted fasting (fast for 16 hours, eat for eight, for instance) every other day or once or twice a week, says Shemek. What that means is Sunday might be a normal day of eating and you'd stop eating by 8 p.m.; then you'd resume eating again on Monday at noon. Essentially, it's like skipping breakfast a few days a week.

Something to keep in mind: According to an article published in December 2015 in the journal Critical Reviews in Food Science and Nutrition, the research is mixed on the effects of skipping breakfast. Some show that eating it is associated with a lower BMI, but there's not consistent evidence in randomized trials that it will cause weight loss. Other research, such as one study published in October 2017 in the Journal of the American College of Cardiology, has linked breakfast skipping with poorer heart health.

This may be easily adaptable to your lifestyle and is more go-with-the-flow, meaning you can make it work even with a schedule that changes week to week. Still, looser approaches may mean more mild benefits.

INTERMITTENT FASTING: BEGINNER'S GUIDE

What it is: Fasting for 16 hours and then only eating within a specific 8-hour window. For example, only eating from noon-8 PM, essentially skipping breakfast. Some people only eat in a 6-hour window, or even a 4-hour window. This is "feasting" and "fasting" parts of your days and the most common form of Intermittent Fasting. It's also my preferred method (4 years running).

Two examples: The top means you are skipping breakfast, the bottom means you are skipping dinner each day:This is an example of an intermittent fasting plan.

You can adjust this window to make it work for your life:

• If you start eating at: 7AM, stop eating and start fasting at 3pm.

• If you start eating at: 11AM, stop eating and start fasting at 7pm.

• If you start eating at: 2PM, stop eating and start fasting at 10pm.

• If you start eating at: 6PM, stop eating and start fasting at 2AM.

INTERMITTENT FASTING 24 HOUR PLAN

Skip two meals one day, where you take 24 hours off from eating. For example, eat on a normal schedule (finishing dinner at 8PM) and then you don't eat again until 8PM the following day. With this plan, you eat your normal 3 meals per day, and then occasionally pick a day to skip breakfast and lunch the next day. If you can only do an 18 hour fast, or a 20 hour fast, or a 22 hour fast – that's okay! Adjust with different time frames and see how your body responds.

Two examples: skipping breakfast and lunch one day of the week, and then another where you skip lunch and dinner one day, two days in a week. This shows another schedule you can try for your intermittent fasting plan.

Note: You can do this once a week, twice a week, or whatever works best for your life and situation.

By the way, both those weekly charts above come from our free Intermittent Fasting

Should I Eat 6 Small Meals a Day?

Should you eat small meals like these, or larger meals broken up by fasting?

There are a few main reasons why diet books recommend six small meals:

When you eat a meal, your body does have to burn extra calories. Just to process that meal. So, the theory is that if you eat all day long with small meals, your body is constantly burning extra calories and your metabolism is firing at optimal capacity, right? Well, that's not true.

Whether you eat 2000 calories spread out throughout the day, or 2000 calories in a small window, your body will burn the same number of calories processing the food.

So, the whole "keep your metabolism firing at optimum capacity by always eating" sounds good in principle, but reality tells a different story.

When you eat smaller meals, you might be less likely to overeat during your regular meals. I can definitely see some truth here, especially for people who struggle with portion control or don't know how much food they should be eating.

However, once you educate yourself and take control of your eating, some might find that eating six times a day is very prohibitive and requires a lot of effort. I know I do.

Also, because you're eating six small meals, I'd argue that you probably never feel "full," and you might be MORE likely to eat extra calories during each snack.

THINGS TO CONSIDER

Fruit is a great and healthy way to break a fasting period. Now that we're through a lot of the science stuff, let's get into the reality of the situation: why should you consider Intermittent Fasting?

Because it can work for your goals. Although we know that not all calories are created equal, caloric restriction plays a central role in weight loss. When you fast, you are also making it easier to restrict your total caloric intake over the course of the week, which can lead to consistent weight loss and maintenance.

Because it simplifies your day. Rather than having to prepare, pack, eat, and time your meals every 2-3 hours, you simply skip a meal or two and only worry about eating food in your eating window. It's one less decision you have to make every day.

It requires less time (and potentially less money). Rather than having to prepare or purchase three to six meals a day, you only need to prepare two meals. Instead of stopping what you're doing six times a day to eat, you simply only have to stop to eat twice. Rather than having to do the dishes six times, you only have to do them twice. Rather than having to purchase six meals a day, you only need to purchase two. It promotes stronger insulin sensitivity and increased growth hormone secretion, two keys for weight loss and muscle gain. Intermittent fasting helps you create a double whammy for weight loss and building a solid physique. It can level up your brain, including positively counteracting conditions like Parkinson's, Alzheimer's, and dementia.

NEGATIVE EFFECTS OF INTERMITTENT FASTING

Intermittent fasting can make you very hungry

In my own experimentation with Intermittent Fasting since 2014, I have found very few negative side effects with Intermittent Fasting. The biggest concern most people have is that Intermittent Fasting will lead to lower energy, focus, and the "holy crap I am hungry" feeling during the fasting period and ruin them. Will fasting make you hangry like this Muppet? Most likely, you will get use to your new eating pattern. People are concerned that they will spend all morning being miserable because they haven't consumed any food, and thus will be miserable at work and ineffective at whatever task it is they are working on.

If you eat breakfast every morning, your body expects to wake up and eat food.

Once you retrain your body to NOT expect food all day every day (or first thing in the morning), these side-effects become less of an issue. In addition, ghrelin (a hormone that makes you hungry is actually lowest in the mornings and decreases after a few hours of not eating too. The hunger pains will naturally pass. Personally, I found this grumpiness subsided after a few days and now my mornings actually energize me.

Intermittent Fasting can change how we look at gaining muscle and losing weight.

Ultimately, this method flies in the face of the typical "bulk and cut" techniques of overeating to build muscle (along with adding a lot of fat) before cutting calories to lose fat (along with some muscle) and settling down at a higher weight.

FAST DIET

The Fast Diet is a low-calorie plan that aims to help followers lose weight – specifically fat – and reduce their risk of a host of chronic diseases by severely limiting calories two days a week. The plan – created by Michael Mosley, a journalist trained as a doctor at the Royal Free Hospital in London, and Mimi Spencer, a journalist and author – mirrors a pattern of eating often referred to as the 5:2 diet: you eat normally for five days of the week and cut your calories to about 25% of normal intake on two nonconsecutive days of the week. Men consume just 600 calories on their two weekly fast days, while women are limited to 500 calories. Those calories should be spent wisely on high-protein foods, such as skinless chicken, nuts and legumes, as well as fruits and veggies with low glycemic loads like strawberries and carrots.

On the other five days of the week, there's no calorie cap, and no food is off-limits. This freedom isn't permission to binge and make up for your two fast days, but it does mean you shouldn't feel guilty about eating a slice of cake. U.S. News experts evaluate the Fast Diet poorly in all rankings, mostly due to its tough-to-follow nature and health risks in some populations.

Low-Calorie Diet

These diets provide far fewer calories than is generally recommended, which leads to weight loss.

In a 2011 study published by the American Association for Cancer Research, researchers at Genesis Prevention Center at University Hospital in South Manchester, England tested the effects of three kinds of diets on 115 women. One diet looked like the Fast Diet (five days of normal eating and two days following a calorie-restricted, low-carb diet each week), another restricted carbs two days a week but had no calorie restrictions and a final group followed a calorie-restricted Mediterranean diet for all seven days of the week.

After four months, participants following the intermittent low-carbohydrate diets lost an average of 9 pounds, while those on the Mediterranean diet lost an average of 5 pounds.

In a randomized trial of 107 overweight or obese premenopausal women, researchers found that participants who followed an intermittent food energy restriction plan (25% restriction two days a week) lost a comparable amount of weight to the participants who followed a continuous energy restriction plan. After six months, participants following the intermittent calorie restriction plan lost an average of 14 pounds each. Results were published in 2011 in the International Journal of Obesity.

A study published in the July 2013 issue of Physiology & Behavior doesn't discuss intermittent-day fasting, but it addresses the concern of overeating after fasting. Researchers at Cornell University either fed breakfast to or withheld breakfast from a group of student volunteers. They found that those who skipped breakfast reported being hungrier than those who ate breakfast. They also ate more at lunch. Still, the amount they ate didn't fully compensate for the missed meal. Volunteers who skipped breakfast consumed 408 fewer calories over the course of the day than those who ate breakfast.

Studies on every-other-day fasting show mixed results. One published in 2010 in the Nutrition Journal suggested that the technique was effective among a group of obese patients. A group of 16 participants ate only one meal – lunch – every other day, and they were limited to about 500 calories. That's the same amount of calories women consume on the Fast Diet's fasting days. On the days when the study participants were not fasting, they were not constrained to any rules. Over the course of eight weeks, the participants lost an average of 12 3/10 pounds.

FAST DIET 2

The fast diet, a form of what's called the 5:2 diet, uses modified intermittent fasting to help people lose weight. Specifically, people following the fast diet eat very few calories (approximately 500 calories for women and 600 calories for men) on two non-consecutive days per week and then eat what they want on the other five days.

Proponents of the diet say it works short-term to help them lose weight, and long-term to keep the weight off. The diet is simple to follow: It involves calorie-counting only on two days per week and doesn't ban any particular types of foods.

However, this can be a difficult diet to stick to, especially at first, since the substantial variation in day-to-day caloric intake may lead to extreme fluctuations in blood sugar (which can affect energy and mood), significant hunger, and possibly other side effects, including headaches. This type of eating plan doesn't teach followers how to eat a healthful diet on the days that they can eat regularly and it's not a healthy diet choice for people with certain health conditions.

What to Eat

Compliant Foods

• Fresh fruit

• Low-fat cottage cheese or yogurt

• Lean chicken

• Salmon, tuna, and other fish

• Steamed vegetables

• Boiled or poached eggs

• Oatmeal

Non-Compliant Foods

• Fried foods

• Red meat

• Cookies, candy, and other sweets

• Sugary drinks (including sweetened coffee and soda)

• Ice cream

• Large portions of any food

When deciding what foods to eat during fasting days, the program recommends consuming foods with a low glycemic index, along with some protein.

The Fast Diet provides numerous suggested menus that add up to 500 or 600 calories per day. For example, breakfast could include oatmeal with skim milk and half a medium pear (307 calories in total) or two poached eggs with one sliced tomato (198 calories). Alternatively, you could have one large boiled egg with half a small grapefruit (130 calories), or a scant half-cup of low-fat cottage cheese, half a sliced pear, and one fresh fig (152 calories).

Dinner could feature salmon with tuna sashimi and broccolini topped with olive oil (341 calories), vegetarian chili (383 calories), chicken stir-fry with vegetables (360 calories), no-carb Caesar salad with chicken, Canadian bacon, grated Parmesan cheese, and romaine lettuce (295 calories), or pesto-topped salmon with baked vegetables (400 calories).

Your choices of what to eat on fasting days will be limited to foods that fit into the low-calorie pattern; a giant slice of chocolate cake (650 calories) or large flavored coffee drink (around 500 calories) are unlikely to fit into your caloric allowance. However, on this diet, you can save those for your non-fasting days.

PROS AND CONS

PROS

SOME DIETS are complicated, with rules about combining foods and timing meals. The fast diet is simple in comparison—you just need to know how to count calories and keep track of which days you're fasting.

The fast diet also allows plenty of food choices. Nothing is expressly forbidden, and in fact, some indulgence is encouraged on non-fasting days. This should help you fight any feelings of deprivation, which can derail a diet.

Finally, there's some scientific backing for intermittent fasting, which has been studied for its effects on longevity. Although the research on it isn't definitive, studies suggest that intermittent fasting could be helpful in improving cardiovascular health and markers of inflammation.

Cons

The fast diet allows you to eat whatever you want, which is a benefit, but also a detriment since it doesn't teach you how to make healthier food choices on your non-fasting days. The book does include multiple recipes, but they're aimed only at your fasting days and so they're extremely low in calories.

In addition, intermittent fasting isn't safe for those with eating disorders, since it could encourage both binge eating and anorexic behavior. It's also not safe for women who are pregnant. And, anyone who's been diagnosed with diabetes and/or heart disease should talk with their doctor before trying the diet, since it may not be the best choice for people with those conditions.

Finally, fasting can be extremely uncomfortable. People who fast often complain of headaches, fatigue, and general malaise. They also may feel light-headed. The fast diet can be difficult to stick with (and potentially unsafe for some people) because of this.

THE DANGERS OF INTERMITTENT FASTING

Intermittent fasting seems to be the new trend swirling among society. Intermittent fasting is a predetermined period that an individual purposely doesn't eat food. There are many different kinds of fasting techniques, just like there are many kinds of diets. From the 12-hour fast to the alternate day fasting, there are many kinds of fasts that are becoming increasingly popular. The thought behind intermittent fasting is that after the body is depleted of carbohydrates, it starts to burn fat around 12-24 hours after starvation so therefore starving the body of food for 12-24 hours will potentially lead to weight loss which can improve health. However, most of the studies done on this topic have been performed on animals over a short period and have measured glucose levels rather than long-term health outcomes. Many argue that intermittent fasting is not necessarily dangerous, but many also agree that intermittent fasting is not safe for everyone. So yes, it is possible to lose calories, fat and weight from this popular diet however it is also possible to just as quickly gain the weight back, develop low energy stores which can result in a depressed mood, problems sleeping and even organ damage if the fasting is extreme. The following are reasons why individuals should avoid intermittent fasting:

You should avoid fasting altogether if you have higher caloric needs

Individuals who are underweight, struggling with weight gain, under 18 years of age, pregnant or who are breastfeeding should not attempt an intermittent fasting diet, as they need sufficient calories on a daily basis for proper development.

You should avoid fasting altogether if you are at risk of an eating disorder

Intermittent fasting has a high association with bulimia nervosa, and as a result, individuals who are susceptible to an eating disorder should not undergo any diet associated with fasting. Risk factors for an eating disorder include having a family member with an eating disorder, perfectionism, impulsivity and mood instability.

You will most likely feel hungry, overeat, become dehydrated, feel tired and be irritable

Intermittent fasting is not for the faint of heart, meaning that even if you are not underweight, you are over 18 years of age, you are not predisposed to an eating disorder, and you are not pregnant or breastfeeding you will most likely have some unwanted side effects.

You will most likely notice your stomach is grumbling during fasting periods, primarily if you are used to constant grazing throughout the day. To avoid these hunger pains during fasting periods, avoid looking at, smelling, or even thinking about food, which can trigger the release of gastric acid into your stomach and make you feel hungry.

Non-fasting days are not days when you can splurge on whatever you want as this can lead to weight gain. Fasting may also lead to an increase in the stress hormone, cortisol, which may lead to even more food cravings. Keep in mind that overeating and binge eating are two common side effects of intermittent fasting.

Intermittent fasting is sometimes associated with dehydration because when you do not eat, sometimes you forget to drink, so it is essential to actively stay hydrated throughout the day by drinking, on average, three liters of water.

You will most likely feel tired because your body is running on less energy than usual, and since fasting can boost stress levels, it can also disrupt your sleep patterns. Therefore it is crucial to adopt a healthy, regular sleep pattern and stick to it so you can feel rested on an everyday basis.

The same biochemistry that regulates mood also regulates appetite with nutrient consumption affecting the activity of neurotransmitters like dopamine and serotonin, which play a role in anxiety and depression.

That means deregulating your appetite may do the same to your mood and therefore you will most likely feel irritable on occasions when you are fasting.

The last piece of advice for individuals who are interested in an intermittent fasting diet it limits your alcohol intake only during eating periods. Do not drink alcohol during or immediately after fasting and even if you drink during your eating periods, keep in mind that drinking alcohol means that you are displacing your opportunity for adequate nutrition

CONCLUSION

It's likely that you'll lose weight if you follow the fast diet—studies show that people don't consume enough extra calories on their non-fasting days to make up for their caloric deficits on their fasting days. There also may be some health benefits to intermittent fasting, although more research is needed.

However, fasting can be hard, and you may feel bad (not to mention quite hungry) on your first few fasting days if you follow this program. In addition, the fast diet may not be safe for people with certain health conditions, including eating disorders, diabetes, and heart disease. And, remember that the fast diet doesn't necessarily focus on healthy food choices.

The Fast Diet says that you shouldn't fast if you're pregnant or underweight, or if you have a history of eating disorders or diabetes, and that you should check with your doctor first if you take medication. The diet also isn't recommended for kids, teens, frail seniors, or anyone who isn't feeling well or has a fever.